CONTENTS

INTRODUCTION

Overview of the Pritikin Diet

The Pritikin Diet is a popular eating plan that emphasizes low-fat, high-fiber, and nutrient-dense foods. It was developed by Nathan Pritikin in the 1970s and has since gained recognition for its potential health benefits. The diet focuses on consuming whole, unprocessed foods and minimizing the intake of saturated fats, cholesterol, and sodium. It is often recommended for individuals looking to improve their overall health, manage weight, and reduce the risk of chronic diseases such as heart disease, hypertension, and diabetes.

The Pritikin Diet primarily consists of fruits, vegetables, whole grains, and lean protein sources such as fish, poultry, and legumes. It encourages the consumption of plant-based foods, including leafy greens, cruciferous vegetables, berries, and nuts. These foods are rich in essential vitamins, minerals, and dietary fiber, which can support digestive health, regulate blood sugar levels, and promote satiety.

One of the key principles of the Pritikin Diet is its focus on reducing the intake of dietary fat, especially saturated and trans fats. These types of fats are commonly found in processed foods, fried foods, and high-fat animal products. By limiting their consumption, the Pritikin Diet aims to lower cholesterol levels and reduce the risk of cardiovascular diseases. Instead, the diet encourages the inclusion of healthy fats, such as those found in avocados, nuts, and seeds, which provide essential fatty acids and contribute to overall well-being.

Another important aspect of the Pritikin Diet is its emphasis on **reducing sodium intake**. High sodium levels can lead to water retention, increased blood pressure, and cardiovascular strain. The diet promotes the use of herbs, spices, and natural seasonings to enhance the flavor of meals without relying on excessive salt. By following these guidelines, individuals can better manage their blood pressure and support heart health.

Explanation of the Health Benefits

The Pritikin Diet offers numerous health benefits due to its emphasis on nutrient-dense foods and overall healthy eating habits. By following this diet plan, individuals may experience:

1. Weight Management: The Pritikin Diet is known for its effectiveness in weight loss and weight management. The focus on whole, unprocessed foods and the restriction of high-calorie, low-nutrient options can help individuals achieve a calorie deficit while still meeting their nutritional needs. Additionally, the high fiber content of the diet promotes feelings of fullness, reducing the likelihood of overeating.

2. Heart Health: The Pritikin Diet is particularly beneficial for heart health due to its emphasis on low-fat, low-cholesterol foods. By reducing the intake of saturated and trans fats, individuals can lower their cholesterol levels, decrease the risk of developing atherosclerosis, and improve overall cardiovascular function. The diet's focus on high-fiber foods, such as fruits, vegetables, and whole grains, can also contribute to lower blood pressure levels and improved heart health.

3. Blood Sugar Control: The Pritikin Diet's emphasis on whole, unprocessed foods and complex carbohydrates can help individuals maintain stable blood sugar levels. The high fiber content of the diet slows down the absorption of glucose, preventing sudden spikes and crashes in blood sugar. This can be particularly beneficial for individuals with diabetes or those at risk of developing the condition.

4. Improved Nutrient Intake: By prioritizing whole, unprocessed foods, the Pritikin Diet ensures that individuals consume a wide range of essential vitamins, minerals, and antioxidants. Fruits and vegetables, in particular, provide an array of micronutrients that support overall health and well-being. The diet also encourages the consumption of lean protein sources and healthy fats, ensuring a well-rounded nutrient intake.

5. Reduced Inflammation: The Pritikin Diet's focus on whole, plant-based foods can help reduce chronic inflammation in the body. Many processed and high-fat foods have been linked to increased inflammation, which is associated with a variety of health conditions, including heart disease, arthritis, and certain cancers. By consuming anti-inflammatory foods, individuals may experience a reduction in inflammation markers and associated health benefits.

Brief History and Background of the Diet

The Pritikin Diet was developed by Nathan Pritikin, an engineer and inventor who had a personal interest in nutrition and health. Pritikin himself had experienced heart disease and was motivated to find a way to improve his own health. Through extensive research and experimentation, he developed an eating plan that focused on whole, unprocessed foods and low-fat, high-fiber choices.

In the 1970s, Nathan Pritikin opened the Pritikin Longevity Center in California, where individuals could learn about and adopt his dietary principles. The center provided a comprehensive program that included education, exercise, and counseling to support overall health and well-being. The Pritikin Diet gained popularity and recognition for its potential to improve heart health and reduce the risk of chronic diseases.

Over the years, the Pritikin Diet has evolved and adapted to incorporate new research and scientific findings. The diet has been endorsed by various health organizations and has been studied extensively for its effectiveness in weight loss, heart disease prevention, and diabetes management. Today, the principles of the Pritikin Diet continue to guide individuals seeking to improve their health through sustainable and nutritious eating habits.

In conclusion, the Pritikin Diet is a low-fat, high-fiber eating plan that promotes whole, unprocessed foods while minimizing the intake of saturated fats, cholesterol, and sodium. It offers a range of health benefits, including weight management, improved heart health, better blood sugar control, enhanced nutrient intake, and reduced inflammation. The diet has a rich history, originating from Nathan Pritikin's personal journey to improve his own health. With its focus on healthy eating habits and long-term well-being, the Pritikin Diet continues to be a popular choice for individuals looking to optimize their health and reduce the risk of chronic diseases.

UNDERSTANDING THE PRITIKIN DIET

The Philosophy behind the Pritikin Diet

The Pritikin Diet is based on the philosophy that by consuming a diet primarily consisting of whole, unprocessed foods, individuals can optimize their health and reduce the risk of chronic diseases. The diet promotes the idea that the human body thrives on a balanced intake of essential nutrients and benefits from the avoidance of excessive saturated fats, cholesterol, and sodium.

The philosophy behind the Pritikin Diet is rooted in the belief that the foods we consume play a significant role in our overall well-being. The diet encourages individuals to prioritize plant-based foods, such as fruits, vegetables, whole grains, and legumes, which provide a rich array of vitamins, minerals, and dietary fiber. By focusing on these nutrient-dense foods, the diet aims to nourish the body and support its optimal functioning.

In addition, the Pritikin Diet promotes a reduction in the consumption of processed and high-fat foods. This is based on the understanding that such foods are often low in nutrients and can contribute to various health issues, including obesity, heart disease, and diabetes. By minimizing the intake of these unhealthy choices, the diet aims to improve overall health outcomes and enhance longevity.

The philosophy behind the Pritikin Diet also emphasizes the importance of lifestyle changes and regular physical activity. It recognizes that a healthy diet alone is not sufficient for achieving optimal health and well-being. Therefore, the diet encourages individuals to incorporate regular exercise into their routine to complement the dietary principles and promote overall vitality.

Principles of the Pritikin Diet

The Pritikin Diet is based on several core principles that guide its approach to nutrition and health:

1. **Emphasis on Whole, Unprocessed Foods:** The diet prioritizes whole, unprocessed foods that are as close

to their natural state as possible. This includes fruits, vegetables, whole grains, legumes, lean protein sources, and healthy fats. By consuming these foods, individuals benefit from their high nutritional content and avoid the additives, preservatives, and excessive processing found in many processed foods.

2. Low-Fat, High-Fiber Choices: The Pritikin Diet promotes a low-fat approach, particularly in relation to saturated and trans fats. These types of fats are often found in animal products and processed foods. Instead, the diet encourages the consumption of high-fiber choices, such as fruits, vegetables, whole grains, and legumes. This combination supports heart health, weight management, and overall well-being.

3. Minimization of Sodium Intake: The diet emphasizes the reduction of sodium intake. Excessive sodium consumption is associated with high blood pressure and an increased risk of cardiovascular diseases. The Pritikin Diet encourages individuals to use natural seasonings, herbs, and spices to flavor their meals, rather than relying on salt.

4. Portion Control: While the focus is on nutrient-dense foods, portion control is also an important aspect of the Pritikin Diet. By being mindful of portion sizes, individuals can maintain a balanced calorie intake and support weight management.

5. Regular Physical Activity: The Pritikin Diet recognizes the importance of regular physical activity in achieving optimal health. It encourages individuals to engage in moderate-intensity exercises, such as walking, swimming, or cycling, for at least 30 minutes a day. Regular exercise complements the dietary principles of the Pritikin Diet and promotes overall well-being.

Scientific Basis and Research Supporting the Diet

The Pritikin Diet has a strong scientific basis, with research supporting its effectiveness in promoting health and reducing the risk of chronic diseases. Multiple studies have examined the impact of the diet on various health outcomes, providing valuable insights into its benefits.

For instance, research has consistently shown that the Pritikin Diet is effective in promoting weight loss and weight management. Studies have demonstrated significant reductions in body weight, body mass index (BMI), and waist circumference among individuals following the diet. This weight loss is often accompanied by improvements in lipid profiles, including reduced total cholesterol, LDL cholesterol, and triglyceride levels.

The Pritikin Diet has also been extensively studied for its effects on heart health. Research has indicated that the diet is associated with lower blood pressure levels, improved endothelial function, and reduced inflammation markers. These factors contribute to a decreased risk of developing heart disease and related complications.

Furthermore, the Pritikin Diet has shown positive effects on blood sugar control and diabetes management. Studies have reported improvements in insulin sensitivity, glycemic control, and HbA1c levels among individuals following the diet. These findings suggest that the diet may be beneficial for individuals with diabetes or those at risk of developing the condition.

Overall, the scientific research supporting the Pritikin Diet demonstrates its potential to improve various health markers and reduce the risk of chronic diseases. The emphasis on whole, unprocessed foods, low-fat choices, and regular physical activity aligns with established principles of healthy eating and lifestyle habits.

In conclusion, the Pritikin Diet is guided by the philosophy that whole, unprocessed foods and healthy lifestyle choices can optimize health and reduce the risk of chronic diseases. The diet's principles focus on nutrient-dense foods, low-fat options, minimized sodium intake, portion control, and regular physical activity. Extensive scientific research supports the effectiveness of the diet in promoting weight loss, improving heart health, managing blood sugar levels, and enhancing overall well-being.

THE PRITIKIN DIET GUIDELINES

Overview of the Food Groups and Their Importance

The Pritikin Diet emphasizes the consumption of various food groups to ensure a well-rounded and balanced intake of nutrients. Here is an overview of the important food groups and their importance within the diet:

1. **Fruits and Vegetables:** These are vital components of the Pritikin Diet. Fruits and vegetables are rich in vitamins, minerals, antioxidants, and dietary fiber. They contribute to overall health, support digestion, and help reduce the risk of chronic diseases.

2. **Whole Grains:** Whole grains provide complex carbohydrates, fiber, and essential nutrients. They are a significant source of sustained energy and promote satiety. Examples of whole grains include brown rice, quinoa, whole wheat bread, and oats.

3. **Legumes:** Legumes, such as beans, lentils, and chickpeas, are excellent sources of plant-based protein, dietary fiber, vitamins, and minerals. They can be used as a substitute for animal protein and contribute to heart health and weight management.

4. **Lean Protein Sources:** The Pritikin Diet encourages the consumption of lean protein sources, including fish (such as salmon and tuna), skinless poultry, and soy products. These provide high-quality protein, omega-3 fatty acids, and essential amino acids while being low in saturated fat.

5. **Healthy Fats:** The diet emphasizes the inclusion of healthy fats, such as those found in avocados, nuts, seeds, and olive oil. These fats are important for brain health, hormone production, and nutrient absorption. However, portion control is essential, as fats are calorie-dense.

6. **Dairy and Dairy Alternatives:** The Pritikin Diet recommends choosing low-fat or non-fat dairy products or plant-based alternatives. These can provide calcium, vitamin D, and protein. It is important to limit the intake of full-fat dairy due to its higher saturated fat content.

7. **Herbs, Spices, and Natural Seasonings:** The Pritikin Diet encourages the use of herbs, spices, and natural seasonings to add flavor to meals without relying on excessive salt, which helps reduce sodium intake.

The inclusion of these food groups in the Pritikin Diet

ensures a diverse and nutrient-rich diet, supporting overall health and well-being.

Recommended Daily Caloric Intake

The recommended daily caloric intake on the Pritikin Diet depends on factors such as age, sex, weight, activity level, and health goals. However, a general guideline for calorie intake is as follows:

1. For Weight Loss: The diet typically recommends a calorie deficit of around 500-1000 calories per day for gradual and sustainable weight loss. This may result in a daily caloric intake ranging from 1200 to 1800 calories, depending on individual needs.

2. For Weight Maintenance: To maintain weight, the daily caloric intake should align with energy expenditure. This can vary between individuals but generally ranges from 1800 to 2200 calories.

It is important to note that these are general recommendations, and individuals should consult with a healthcare professional or registered dietitian to determine their specific calorie needs based on their unique circumstances.

Macronutrient Distribution: Carbohydrates, Proteins, and Fats

The Pritikin Diet promotes a balanced macronutrient distribution that focuses on high-quality carbohydrates, adequate protein, and limited fats. Here is a breakdown of the recommended macronutrient distribution:

1. **Carbohydrates:** The Pritikin Diet emphasizes complex carbohydrates, which are found in fruits, vegetables, whole grains, and legumes. These should form the foundation of the diet and provide approximately 50-60% of daily caloric intake. Complex carbohydrates offer sustained energy, fiber, and essential nutrients.

2. **Proteins:** The diet recommends consuming moderate amounts of lean protein sources, such as fish, poultry, legumes, and soy products. Protein intake should make up around 15-20% of daily caloric intake. Adequate protein is important for muscle maintenance, repair, and overall body functioning.

3. **Fats:** The Pritikin Diet recommends limiting the intake of fats, particularly saturated and trans fats. Healthy fats, such as those from avocados, nuts, seeds, and olive oil, should be consumed in moderation. Fats should constitute approximately 20-30% of daily caloric intake. Portion control is crucial due to the higher calorie density of fats.

The emphasis on complex carbohydrates and adequate protein, along with controlled fat intake, supports overall health, weight management, and reduced risk of chronic diseases.

List of Allowed and Restricted Foods

The Pritikin Diet provides guidance on allowed and restricted foods to support healthy eating choices. Here is a general overview:

Allowed Foods:

- Fruits and vegetables (including fresh, frozen, or canned without added sugars)
- Whole grains (such as brown rice, quinoa, oats, whole wheat bread)
- Legumes (beans, lentils, chickpeas)
- Lean protein sources (skinless poultry, fish, soy products)
- Low-fat or non-fat dairy products or dairy alternatives
- Healthy fats (avocados, nuts, seeds, olive oil)
- Herbs, spices, and natural seasonings for flavoring

Restricted Foods:

- Processed and refined foods (such as white bread, white rice, sugary cereals)
- High-fat meats (fatty cuts of beef, pork, processed meats)
- Full-fat dairy products

- High-fat snack foods (chips, fried foods)
- Added sugars and sugary beverages
- Foods high in sodium and excessive salt

The Pritikin Diet encourages individuals to prioritize whole, unprocessed foods and make mindful choices that support their health goals.

Importance of Portion Control

Portion control is a key aspect of the Pritikin Diet. While the focus is on nutrient-dense foods, it is crucial to consume them in appropriate quantities. Here's why portion control is important:

1. **Calorie Management:** Controlling portion sizes helps manage overall calorie intake. Even healthy foods can contribute to weight gain if consumed in excess. By practicing portion control, individuals can maintain a balanced calorie intake that aligns with their health goals.

2. **Satiety and Fullness:** Proper portion sizes help ensure satiety and prevent overeating. By eating appropriate portions, individuals can feel satisfied without consuming excess calories.

3. **Balanced Macronutrient Intake:** Portion control ensures a balanced distribution of macronutrients. By controlling portion sizes of carbohydrates, proteins, and fats, individuals can achieve the desired macronutrient ratios and support overall health.

4. **Consistency and Sustainability:** Portion control promotes consistency and sustainability in healthy eating habits. It allows individuals to enjoy a variety of foods while maintaining a balanced approach.

Practicing portion control alongside the principles of the Pritikin Diet helps individuals maintain a healthy weight, manage portion sizes, and develop mindful eating habits.

In summary, the Pritikin Diet encourages the consumption of various food groups, including fruits, vegetables, whole grains, legumes, lean proteins, healthy fats, and low-fat dairy or dairy alternatives. Portion control is emphasized to manage calorie intake and support weight management. The diet focuses on a balanced macronutrient distribution, with complex carbohydrates forming the majority, followed by adequate protein and controlled fat intake. By following the allowed and restricted food guidelines and practicing portion control, individuals can achieve a balanced and nutrient-rich diet that supports their health and well-being.

KEY COMPONENTS OF THE PRITIKIN DIET

High-Fiber Foods and Their Benefits

High-fiber foods play a crucial role in the Pritikin Diet and offer numerous benefits for overall health. Here are some of the benefits associated with consuming high-fiber foods:

1. **Digestive Health:** Fiber promotes healthy digestion by adding bulk to the stool and supporting regular bowel movements. It helps prevent constipation and promotes a healthy gut microbiome.

2. **Weight Management:** High-fiber foods tend to be more filling, which can help with appetite control and weight management. Fiber-rich foods require more chewing and take longer to digest, providing a greater sense of satiety and reducing the likelihood of overeating.

3. **Blood Sugar Control:** Fiber slows down the

absorption of sugar into the bloodstream, helping to stabilize blood sugar levels. This is particularly beneficial for individuals with diabetes or those at risk of developing the condition.

4. **Heart Health:** High-fiber foods, especially soluble fiber, can help lower cholesterol levels by reducing the absorption of dietary cholesterol. This, in turn, can reduce the risk of heart disease and stroke.

5. **Reduced Risk of Chronic Diseases:** A diet high in fiber has been associated with a lower risk of developing various chronic diseases, including obesity, type 2 diabetes, certain types of cancer (such as colorectal cancer), and cardiovascular diseases.

Some examples of high-fiber foods include fruits, vegetables, whole grains, legumes, nuts, and seeds. By incorporating these foods into the diet, individuals can reap the numerous benefits of a high-fiber intake.

Whole Grains and Their Role in the Diet

Whole grains play a vital role in the Pritikin Diet due to their nutritional value and health benefits. Here's why whole grains are important:

1. **Nutrient-Rich:** Whole grains contain the entire grain kernel, including the bran, germ, and endosperm. This means they retain valuable nutrients such as fiber, B vitamins, minerals (like

iron and magnesium), and antioxidants.

2. **Dietary Fiber:** Whole grains are excellent sources of dietary fiber, both soluble and insoluble. Fiber aids digestion, promotes feelings of fullness, and supports healthy bowel movements.

3. **Sustained Energy:** The complex carbohydrates found in whole grains provide a steady release of energy, keeping blood sugar levels stable and providing lasting fuel for the body.

4. **Heart Health:** Whole grains have been associated with a reduced risk of heart disease. The fiber, antioxidants, and other compounds in whole grains help lower cholesterol levels, decrease blood pressure, and support overall cardiovascular health.

5. **Weight Management:** The high fiber content of whole grains contributes to satiety, helping individuals feel fuller for longer. This can aid in weight management by reducing the likelihood of overeating.

Some examples of whole grains include brown rice, quinoa, oats, whole wheat, barley, buckwheat, and whole grain bread and pasta. When incorporating grains into the diet, choosing whole grain options provides a range of health benefits and ensures a nutrient-rich eating plan.

Lean Proteins and Their Sources

Lean proteins are an essential component of the Pritikin

Diet. These proteins provide important amino acids for muscle maintenance, repair, and overall body functioning. Here are some lean protein sources recommended on the diet:

1. **Poultry:** Skinless chicken breast and turkey breast are lean sources of protein. They provide high-quality protein without excessive saturated fat. It's important to choose lean cuts and avoid frying or using high-fat cooking methods.

2. **Fish:** Fatty fish like salmon, mackerel, trout, and sardines are rich in omega-3 fatty acids, which have numerous health benefits. White fish such as cod, haddock, and tilapia are also lean protein options.

3. **Legumes:** Legumes, including beans, lentils, and chickpeas, are excellent plant-based sources of protein. They are also high in fiber, vitamins, and minerals. Legumes can be incorporated into soups, stews, salads, or used as a meat substitute in various recipes.

4. **Soy Products:** Tofu, tempeh, edamame, and soy milk are examples of soy-based products that provide complete protein. Soy products are suitable for vegetarians and vegans and offer versatility in cooking.

5. **Egg Whites:** Egg whites are a low-fat, high-protein option. They can be used in omelettes, scrambled eggs, or added to baked goods for a protein boost.

When choosing lean proteins, it is important to prepare them using healthy cooking methods such as grilling, baking, steaming, or sautéing with minimal added fats.

Healthy Fats and Their Importance

Healthy fats are an essential part of the Pritikin Diet, providing essential nutrients and supporting various bodily functions. Here's why healthy fats are important:

1. **Nutrient Absorption:** Fats play a crucial role in the absorption of fat-soluble vitamins (vitamins A, D, E, and K). These vitamins require the presence of dietary fat to be effectively absorbed by the body.

2. **Brain Health:** The brain relies on healthy fats for optimal functioning. Omega-3 fatty acids, found in fatty fish, walnuts, flaxseeds, and chia seeds, are particularly beneficial for brain health and may help reduce the risk of cognitive decline.

3. **Cellular Function:** Fats are integral components of cell membranes and play a role in maintaining cell structure and function.

4. **Hormone Production:** Certain fats are necessary for the production of hormones in the body. They are involved in regulating various bodily processes, including metabolism, growth, and reproductive health.

5. **Heart Health:** Healthy fats, such as monounsaturated and polyunsaturated fats, can

help improve blood cholesterol levels, reduce inflammation, and lower the risk of heart disease. Some sources of healthy fats include avocados, nuts (such as almonds, walnuts, and pistachios), seeds (such as flaxseeds and chia seeds), olives, olive oil, and fatty fish. While healthy fats are important, portion control is crucial as they are calorie-dense.

Incorporating Fruits and Vegetables

The Pritikin Diet emphasizes the incorporation of fruits and vegetables due to their nutrient density and health benefits. Here's why fruits and vegetables are important in the diet:

1. **Nutrient-Rich:** Fruits and vegetables are packed with essential vitamins, minerals, antioxidants, and dietary fiber. They provide a wide range of nutrients necessary for overall health and well-being.

2. **Disease Prevention:** A diet rich in fruits and vegetables has been associated with a reduced risk of chronic diseases, including heart disease, certain cancers, and age-related macular degeneration.

3. **Fiber Content:** Fruits and vegetables are excellent sources of dietary fiber, both soluble and insoluble. Fiber aids in digestion, supports a healthy gut, and promotes feelings of fullness.

4. **Hydration and Electrolyte Balance:** Many fruits and vegetables have high water content, contributing to hydration and electrolyte balance. They can help replenish fluids and provide essential minerals, such as potassium.

5. **Variety and Flavour:** Fruits and vegetables offer a wide range of colours, textures, and flavours. Incorporating a variety of fruits and vegetables into meals can make the diet more enjoyable, diverse, and satisfying.

The Pritikin Diet encourages individuals to include a variety of fruits and vegetables in their daily meals and snacks. Fresh, frozen, or canned options without added sugars or excess sodium are all suitable choices. Aim to fill half your plate with fruits and vegetables to ensure a balanced and nutritious diet.

In conclusion, the Pritikin Diet promotes the consumption of high-fiber foods, including fruits, vegetables, whole grains, legumes, nuts, and seeds. Lean proteins, such as poultry, fish, legumes, and soy products, provide essential amino acids. Healthy fats from sources like avocados, nuts, seeds, and olive oil are incorporated in moderation. By including a variety of fruits and vegetables, individuals can ensure nutrient diversity and enjoy the health benefits associated with these food groups.

MEAL PLANNING ON THE PRITIKIN DIET

Sample Meal Plans for Breakfast, Lunch, and Dinner

Here are some sample meal plans for each main meal of the day on the Pritikin Diet:

Breakfast:

- Option 1: Oatmeal topped with mixed berries, sliced almonds, and a drizzle of honey. Serve with a side of Greek yogurt.

- Option 2: Vegetable omelette made with egg whites, spinach, tomatoes, and mushrooms. Enjoy with a slice of whole grain toast.

- Option 3: Quinoa breakfast bowl with diced fruit, chopped nuts, and a sprinkle of cinnamon.

Lunch:

- Option 1: Grilled chicken breast served on a bed of mixed greens, cherry tomatoes, cucumber slices, and a light vinaigrette dressing.

- Option 2: Lentil salad with mixed vegetables, diced bell peppers, and a lemon herb dressing.
- Option 3: Whole grain wrap filled with lean turkey breast, avocado, lettuce, and tomato. Enjoy with a side of vegetable sticks.

Dinner:

- Option 1: Baked salmon seasoned with herbs and served with steamed broccoli and quinoa.
- Option 2: Stir-fried tofu and mixed vegetables in a light soy sauce. Serve over brown rice.
- Option 3: Grilled chicken skewers with bell peppers and onions. Enjoy with a side of roasted sweet potatoes and a green salad.

Remember to adjust portion sizes based on your individual calorie needs and consult with a healthcare professional or nutritionist for personalized guidance.

Snack Ideas and Guidelines

Snacks can be an important part of the Pritikin Diet to help keep hunger at bay and maintain energy levels throughout the day. Here are some snack ideas that align with the principles of the diet:

- Fresh fruit, such as apple slices with almond butter or a banana

- Raw vegetable sticks with hummus or Greek yogurt dip
- Mixed nuts and seeds (in moderation)
- Greek yogurt with berries
- Whole grain crackers with low-fat cheese or avocado slices
- Hard-boiled eggs
- Homemade smoothies using fruits, vegetables, and a source of protein like Greek yogurt or tofu
- Air-popped popcorn sprinkled with herbs or nutritional yeast

Remember to practice portion control even with snacks to maintain a balanced calorie intake. It can be helpful to pre-portion snacks into individual servings to avoid overeating.

Strategies for Dining Out or Traveling While on the Diet

Maintaining the Pritikin Diet while dining out or traveling may require some planning and preparation. Here are some strategies to help you stay on track:

1. **Research and Choose Wisely:** Before dining out, review the menu online if available. Look for dishes that feature lean proteins, vegetables, and whole grains. Avoid fried and heavily sauced options. Request modifications, such as dressing

on the side or steamed vegetables instead of fries.

2. **Ask Questions:** Don't hesitate to ask the waitstaff about ingredients, cooking methods, or any special requests you have. Most restaurants are accommodating and can provide healthier alternatives or adjustments.

3. **Portion Control:** Restaurant portions are often larger than necessary. Consider sharing a dish with a dining partner or ask for a to-go box to pack up leftovers before you start eating.

4. **Smart Swaps:** Make healthier substitutions when possible. Opt for grilled or steamed options instead of fried. Choose whole grain options like brown rice or whole wheat bread instead of refined grains.

5. **Stay Hydrated:** Keep yourself hydrated while traveling by carrying a refillable water bottle. Limit sugary drinks and opt for water, unsweetened tea, or sparkling water instead.

6. **Pack Snacks:** When traveling, pack nutritious snacks like fresh fruit, cut vegetables, nuts, or whole grain crackers to have on hand. This helps you avoid relying on unhealthy options available during travel.

Tips for Meal Prepping

Meal prepping can be a helpful strategy to stay on track with the Pritikin Diet and save time during the week. Here are some tips to make meal prepping easier:

1. **Plan your meals:** Take some time each week to

plan your meals and create a shopping list. This ensures you have all the ingredients needed for your meals.

2. **Batch cooking:** Prepare larger quantities of staple items like whole grains, lean proteins, and roasted vegetables that can be used in multiple meals throughout the week. This saves time and allows for easy assembly of meals.

3. **Divide and store:** Portion out meals into individual containers for easy grab-and-go options. Store them in the fridge or freezer depending on your meal plan for the week.

4. **Pre-cut and wash:** Wash and cut vegetables and fruits in advance, so they are ready to be used in salads, stir-fries, or snacks. This saves time and encourages healthier choices.

5. **Utilize kitchen gadgets:** Invest in kitchen gadgets like a slow cooker or an Instant Pot that can help simplify meal preparation. These appliances allow for hands-off cooking and can be used for batch cooking as well.

6. **Experiment with flavours:** Prepare different marinades, dressings, or spice mixes to add variety and enhance the flavours of your meals throughout the week.

Remember to practice proper food safety guidelines when meal prepping, such as storing perishable items at the correct temperature and consuming meals within a safe timeframe.

By incorporating these strategies, you can make meal prepping a breeze and ensure that you have nutritious meals readily available throughout the week.

MANAGING WEIGHT ON THE PRITIKIN DIET

How the Diet Supports Weight Loss

The Pritikin Diet is known for its effectiveness in supporting weight loss. Here's how the diet helps in achieving weight loss goals:

1. **Calorie Control:** The Pritikin Diet promotes calorie control by focusing on nutrient-dense, low-calorie foods. By incorporating high-fiber fruits and vegetables, whole grains, lean proteins, and healthy fats, individuals can feel satisfied while consuming fewer calories.

2. **High-Fiber Intake:** The diet emphasizes high-fiber foods, which contribute to feelings of fullness and promote satiety. Fiber-rich foods take longer to digest, keeping you satisfied for longer periods and reducing the tendency to overeat or snack on unhealthy options.

3. **Balanced Macronutrient Ratio:** The Pritikin Diet maintains a balanced distribution of macronutrients. By including an adequate amount of carbohydrates, lean proteins, and healthy fats, the diet provides the necessary nutrients while promoting weight loss.

4. **Low in Added Sugars and Refined Grains:** The diet discourages the consumption of added sugars and refined grains, which are often high in calories and offer little nutritional value. By reducing these empty calorie sources, individuals can better manage their weight.

5. **Healthy Fat Choices:** The diet encourages the consumption of healthy fats from sources such as nuts, seeds, avocados, and olive oil. These fats provide essential nutrients and promote feelings of satisfaction, helping to control overall calorie intake.

6. **Hydration:** Adequate hydration is emphasized in the Pritikin Diet. Drinking plenty of water can help manage hunger and prevent overeating. It also supports overall health and well-being.

By following the principles of the Pritikin Diet, individuals can create a calorie deficit, promote satiety, and make healthier food choices, all of which contribute to weight loss.

Strategies for Portion Control and Mindful Eating

Portion control and mindful eating are important aspects of the Pritikin Diet. Here are some strategies to help with portion control and develop mindful eating habits:

1. **Use Smaller Plates and Bowls:** Using smaller plates and bowls can create an illusion of a fuller plate, helping to control portion sizes and prevent overeating.

2. **Measure and Weigh Food:** Initially, it can be helpful to measure or weigh food to become aware of appropriate portion sizes. This practice enables you to estimate portions more accurately over time.

3. **Practice Mindful Eating:** Pay attention to the sensations of eating, such as the taste, texture, and smell of food. Slow down while eating, chew thoroughly, and savour each bite. Mindful eating helps you tune in to your body's hunger and fullness cues, preventing overeating.

4. **Eat Without Distractions:** Avoid eating in front of the TV or while working on your computer or phone. Engaging in mindful eating means being fully present with your meal and enjoying the eating experience.

5. **Listen to Your Body:** Learn to recognize your body's hunger and fullness signals. Eat when you're physically hungry and stop eating when you're comfortably full. It's important to eat until satisfied, not overly stuffed.

6. **Plan Balanced Meals:** Plan your meals in advance to ensure they include a balance of nutrients,

such as lean proteins, whole grains, vegetables, and healthy fats. This helps you create satisfying meals that support portion control.

By practicing portion control and mindful eating, individuals can develop a healthier relationship with food, improve their eating habits, and achieve their weight loss goals.

Incorporating Physical Activity into the Diet Plan

Physical activity is a crucial component of the Pritikin Diet for overall health and weight management. Here are some strategies to incorporate physical activity into your diet plan:

1. **Choose Activities You Enjoy:** Engage in physical activities that you enjoy and look forward to. This could be brisk walking, cycling, swimming, dancing, or any other form of exercise that gets your heart rate up.

2. **Aim for Regular Exercise:** Strive to engage in moderate-intensity aerobic exercise for at least 150 minutes per week. This can be spread out over several days and can include activities like brisk walking, jogging, or cycling.

3. **Strength Training:** Incorporate strength training exercises at least two days a week. This helps build lean muscle mass, which can increase metabolism

and support weight loss.

4. **Stay Active Throughout the Day:** Find opportunities to move more throughout the day. Take the stairs instead of the elevator, go for short walks during breaks, or engage in household chores that require physical effort.

5. **Consider Group Activities:** Joining exercise classes, sports teams, or fitness groups can provide social support and make physical activity more enjoyable.

6. **Track Your Progress:** Keep a record of your exercise sessions, noting the duration, intensity, and type of activity. This can help you monitor your progress and stay motivated.

Remember to consult with a healthcare professional before starting any exercise program, especially if you have any underlying health conditions.

Monitoring Progress and Setting Realistic Goals

Monitoring progress and setting realistic goals are essential for success on the Pritikin Diet. Here are some tips to help you stay on track:

1. **Track Your Food Intake:** Keep a food diary or use a mobile app to track your daily food intake. This helps create awareness of your eating habits and allows you to identify areas for improvement.

2. **Weigh and Measure:** Regularly weigh yourself and measure your body to track changes in

weight, body fat percentage, or inches lost. However, it's important to remember that weight is not the only measure of success. Focus on overall well-being and improvements in energy levels and fitness.

3. **Celebrate Non-Scale Victories:** Acknowledge and celebrate non-scale victories such as increased energy, improved sleep, better mood, or reduced reliance on medication. These achievements reflect the positive impact of the diet on your overall health.

4. **Set Realistic Goals:** Set achievable, realistic goals that are specific, measurable, attainable, relevant, and time-bound (SMART). Breaking down long-term goals into smaller milestones makes them more manageable and keeps you motivated.

5. **Stay Accountable:** Share your goals with a friend, family member, or a support group. Having someone to be accountable to can provide encouragement and help you stay committed.

6. **Regular Assessments:** Schedule regular check-ins with a healthcare professional or nutritionist to assess your progress, receive guidance, and make any necessary adjustments to your diet and exercise plan.

Remember that weight loss is a journey, and everyone's progress may vary. Be patient, stay consistent, and focus on long-term sustainable changes rather than quick fixes.

By monitoring your progress and setting realistic goals,

you can stay motivated and track the positive changes that come with following the Pritikin Diet and incorporating physical activity into your lifestyle.

ADDRESSING COMMON CONCERNS AND CHALLENGES

Overcoming Cravings and Managing Hunger

Cravings and managing hunger can be challenges when following the Pritikin Diet. Here are some strategies to help overcome cravings and manage hunger effectively:

1. **Stay Hydrated:** Sometimes, thirst can be mistaken for hunger. Stay hydrated by drinking plenty of water throughout the day. Drinking a glass of water before meals can help you feel fuller and reduce the likelihood of overeating.

2. **Include Protein and Fiber:** Protein and fiber-rich foods are known to promote satiety and help manage hunger. Include lean sources of protein, such as poultry, fish, legumes, and tofu, in your

meals. Fiber-rich foods like fruits, vegetables, whole grains, and legumes can also help keep you feeling fuller for longer.

3. **Plan Balanced Meals:** Ensure that your meals are well-balanced and include a combination of complex carbohydrates, proteins, and healthy fats. This helps provide sustained energy and keeps you satisfied until your next meal.

4. **Snack Smart:** Opt for healthy snacks that are low in calories but provide satiety. Choose snacks that contain protein, fiber, and healthy fats, such as Greek yogurt, raw nuts and seeds, or vegetable sticks with hummus.

5. **Mindful Eating:** Practice mindful eating techniques, such as eating slowly, chewing thoroughly, and savoring each bite. Pay attention to your body's hunger and fullness cues to prevent overeating.

6. **Distract Yourself:** When cravings strike, distract yourself by engaging in a non-food related activity. Go for a walk, read a book, or engage in a hobby to shift your focus away from food.

7. **Manage Stress:** Stress can contribute to cravings and emotional eating. Find healthy ways to manage stress, such as practicing relaxation techniques, exercise, or engaging in activities you enjoy.

Remember that cravings and hunger are natural sensations, and it's important to listen to your body's needs while making healthy choices that align with the principles of the Pritikin Diet.

Dealing with Social Situations and Dining Out

Social situations and dining out can present challenges when following the Pritikin Diet. Here are some strategies to navigate these situations:

1. **Plan Ahead:** Before attending social events or dining out, plan your approach. Look up the menu in advance and identify healthier options that align with the Pritikin Diet. If possible, suggest dining at a restaurant that offers healthier choices.

2. **Communicate Your Needs:** Don't hesitate to communicate your dietary preferences and needs to your host or the restaurant staff. Most establishments are willing to accommodate special requests, such as dressing on the side, steamed vegetables instead of fries, or grilled instead of fried preparations.

3. **Portion Control:** Be mindful of portion sizes when dining out. Restaurant servings are often larger than necessary. Consider sharing a dish with a friend, ordering an appetizer as a main course, or asking for a to-go box to pack up leftovers.

4. **Choose Wisely:** Opt for healthier options on the menu. Look for dishes that feature lean proteins, vegetables, whole grains, and minimal added fats or sugars. Avoid dishes that are deep-fried, heavily sauced, or loaded with cheese.

5. **Be Mindful of Beverages:** Alcoholic and sugary beverages can contribute a significant amount of calories. Choose water, unsweetened tea, or sparkling water instead. If you choose to drink alcohol, do so in moderation and opt for lower-calorie options like light beer or wine.

6. **Focus on Enjoyment:** Shift the focus of social gatherings from solely food to the company and conversation. Engage in enjoyable activities that don't revolve around eating, such as taking a walk, playing games, or participating in group activities.

Remember that occasional indulgences are part of a balanced lifestyle. If you do choose to enjoy a treat or a less healthy option, do so in moderation and return to your regular healthy eating habits.

Potential Nutrient Deficiencies and Supplementation

The Pritikin Diet emphasizes whole, nutrient-dense foods, which generally provide the necessary nutrients for overall health. However, it's important to be mindful of potential nutrient deficiencies that may arise due to certain dietary restrictions. Here are some key nutrients to consider:

1. **Vitamin B12:** The Pritikin Diet is primarily plant-based and may be low in vitamin B12, which is mainly found in animal products. Consider taking

a B12 supplement or consuming foods fortified with B12, such as plant-based milks or cereals.

2. **Calcium:** While the Pritikin Diet promotes calcium-rich foods like non-fat dairy products, if you follow a dairy-free version of the diet, you may need to pay attention to calcium intake. Include calcium-rich plant-based sources such as fortified plant milks, tofu, leafy green vegetables, and almonds. Calcium supplements may be considered if needed.

3. **Omega-3 Fatty Acids:** Although the Pritikin Diet includes sources of omega-3 fatty acids like walnuts, flaxseeds, and chia seeds, some individuals may benefit from additional supplementation, especially if they don't consume fish or seafood. Consider incorporating algae-based omega-3 supplements or consulting with a healthcare professional for personalized advice.

4. **Iron:** Plant-based sources of iron are included in the Pritikin Diet, such as legumes, leafy green vegetables, and fortified whole grains. However, the iron from plant-based sources is not as easily absorbed as iron from animal products. To enhance iron absorption, include vitamin C-rich foods like citrus fruits or peppers in your meals.

It's important to consult with a healthcare professional or registered dietitian who can assess your individual nutrient needs and provide personalized recommendations for supplementation if necessary.

Adjusting the Diet for Specific Health Conditions

The Pritikin Diet can be adapted to accommodate specific health conditions or dietary needs. Here are a few examples:

1. **Diabetes:** The Pritikin Diet is suitable for individuals with diabetes. It focuses on low-glycemic index foods, promotes balanced meals, and encourages portion control. However, if you have diabetes, it's essential to monitor your blood sugar levels regularly and work with a healthcare professional or registered dietitian to tailor the diet to your specific needs.

2. **High Blood Pressure:** The Pritikin Diet is beneficial for individuals with high blood pressure. It emphasizes a low-sodium intake by avoiding processed foods and reducing added salt. It also promotes a high intake of fruits, vegetables, whole grains, and lean proteins, which are all associated with blood pressure management.

3. **Cholesterol Management:** The Pritikin Diet is effective in reducing cholesterol levels. It focuses on consuming foods low in saturated and trans fats while emphasizing high-fiber foods, whole grains, and lean proteins. It also discourages the consumption of cholesterol-rich foods like red meat and full-fat dairy products.

4. **Gastrointestinal Disorders:** Individuals with gastrointestinal disorders, such as irritable bowel syndrome (IBS) or inflammatory bowel disease (IBD), may need to make some modifications to the Pritikin Diet. Working with a healthcare professional or registered dietitian can help tailor the diet to meet specific needs, such as identifying trigger foods or incorporating low-FODMAP options.

It's crucial to consult with a healthcare professional or registered dietitian to ensure that any adjustments to the Pritikin Diet are suitable for your specific health condition and dietary requirements. They can provide personalized guidance and support to help you achieve your health goals.

LIFESTYLE FACTORS AND LONG-TERM SUSTAINABILITY

Stress Management and Its Impact on Health

Stress management plays a crucial role in maintaining overall health and well-being. Chronic stress can have negative effects on both physical and mental health. Here are some strategies to manage stress effectively:

1. **Relaxation Techniques:** Practice relaxation techniques such as deep breathing exercises, meditation, or yoga to help reduce stress levels. These techniques can promote a sense of calm and relaxation.

2. **Physical Activity:** Engaging in regular physical activity is not only beneficial for physical health but also for stress reduction. Exercise releases endorphins, which are natural mood boosters. Incorporate activities like walking, jogging, swimming, or dancing into your routine.

3. **Time Management:** Prioritize tasks and create a schedule that allows for a balanced lifestyle. Avoid overloading yourself with responsibilities and learn to delegate when necessary. Effective time management can help reduce feelings of overwhelm.

4. **Healthy Coping Mechanisms:** Find healthy ways to cope with stress rather than turning to unhealthy habits such as overeating or excessive alcohol consumption. Engage in activities you enjoy, spend time with loved ones, or pursue hobbies and interests.

5. **Social Support:** Seek support from friends, family, or support groups. Sharing your feelings and experiences with others can provide comfort and help you gain perspective.

6. **Self-Care:** Make self-care a priority. Engage in activities that promote relaxation and rejuvenation, such as taking baths, reading, listening to music, or practicing mindfulness.

Remember that managing stress is an ongoing process, and different techniques work for different individuals. Find what works best for you and incorporate stress management strategies into your daily routine.

Importance of Regular Exercise and Physical Activity

Regular exercise and physical activity are vital components

of a healthy lifestyle. Here are some reasons why exercise is important:

1. **Weight Management:** Regular exercise helps burn calories and maintain a healthy weight. It promotes fat loss, preserves lean muscle mass, and boosts metabolism.

2. **Cardiovascular Health:** Exercise strengthens the heart and improves cardiovascular health. It can help reduce the risk of heart disease, high blood pressure, and stroke.

3. **Mental Well-being:** Exercise has a positive impact on mental health. It releases endorphins, which can improve mood, reduce stress and anxiety, and promote better sleep.

4. **Bone and Muscle Health:** Weight-bearing exercises, such as walking or strength training, help maintain bone density and prevent conditions like osteoporosis. Strength training also helps build and maintain muscle strength.

5. **Improved Energy Levels:** Regular physical activity increases energy levels and reduces fatigue. It enhances circulation and oxygen delivery to the body, resulting in increased vitality.

6. **Disease Prevention:** Exercise plays a crucial role in preventing chronic diseases such as type 2 diabetes, certain types of cancer, and metabolic syndrome.

It's important to find physical activities that you enjoy and incorporate them into your routine. Aim for a combination of aerobic exercises, strength training, and flexibility exercises for a well-rounded fitness regimen.

Sleep and Its Role in Supporting Overall Well-being

Quality sleep is essential for overall health and well-being. Here's why sleep is important and some strategies to improve sleep quality:

1. **Rest and Recovery:** Sleep allows the body and mind to rest and recover from daily activities. It promotes physical repair, supports immune function, and helps regulate hormones.

2. **Mental Health:** Sufficient sleep is crucial for mental health and emotional well-being. Lack of sleep can contribute to mood swings, irritability, and increased stress levels.

3. **Cognitive Function:** Sleep is essential for optimal cognitive function, including memory consolidation, attention span, and problem-solving abilities. It enhances learning and creativity.

4. **Energy and Productivity:** Quality sleep improves energy levels, concentration, and productivity throughout the day. It allows you to perform daily tasks more effectively.

5. **Healthy Weight Management:** Lack of sleep can disrupt appetite-regulating hormones, leading to

increased cravings and a higher risk of weight gain and obesity.

To improve sleep quality:

1. **Establish a Routine:** Create a regular sleep schedule by going to bed and waking up at consistent times, even on weekends.

2. **Create a Sleep-friendly Environment:** Ensure your sleep environment is dark, quiet, and cool. Use blackout curtains, earplugs, or white noise machines if necessary.

3. **Limit Screen Time:** Avoid electronic devices and stimulating activities before bedtime. The blue light emitted by screens can interfere with sleep.

4. **Relaxation Techniques:** Practice relaxation techniques such as deep breathing, meditation, or gentle stretching before bed to calm the mind and body.

5. **Avoid Stimulants:** Limit or avoid caffeine, nicotine, and alcohol, especially close to bedtime, as they can disrupt sleep patterns.

6. **Create a Bedtime Ritual:** Establish a relaxing routine before bed, such as reading a book, taking a warm bath, or listening to soothing music.

Prioritizing sleep as part of your healthy lifestyle is crucial for overall well-being and should not be overlooked.

Strategies for Maintaining the Pritikin Diet in the Long Term

Maintaining the Pritikin Diet in the long term requires commitment and sustainable habits. Here are some strategies to help you stay on track:

1. **Education and Planning:** Continue to educate yourself about the principles and benefits of the Pritikin Diet. Stay updated on new recipes, meal ideas, and nutritional information. Plan your meals in advance to ensure you have nutritious options available.

2. **Gradual Transition:** If you find it challenging to make sudden dietary changes, consider transitioning gradually. Start by incorporating more whole foods, fruits, vegetables, and whole grains into your diet while gradually reducing processed foods and added sugars.

3. **Variety and Flexibility:** Embrace variety in your meals to prevent boredom. Experiment with different fruits, vegetables, whole grains, and lean proteins. Be flexible and adaptable, allowing for occasional indulgences or modifications when dining out or attending social events.

4. **Social Support:** Seek support from family, friends, or online communities following a similar dietary approach. Share your experiences, challenges, and successes. Having a support network can provide motivation and encouragement.

5. **Regular Shopping and Meal Prep:** Plan your grocery shopping and meal prep to ensure you have healthy ingredients readily available. Batch-cook meals, portion them, and store them in the

fridge or freezer for convenient and nutritious options throughout the week.

6. **Focus on Health Benefits:** Remind yourself of the health benefits you've experienced or are working towards by following the Pritikin Diet. Focus on improved energy levels, weight management, better blood pressure or cholesterol control, and overall well-being.

7. **Regular Self-Assessment:** Periodically evaluate your progress and reassess your goals. Monitor how the diet is working for you and make adjustments as needed. Celebrate your achievements and use setbacks as opportunities to learn and grow.

Remember that the Pritikin Diet is not just a temporary solution but a long-term approach to healthy eating and living. By adopting sustainable habits and incorporating the principles of the diet into your lifestyle, you can reap the benefits and maintain your health and well-being in the long run.

SUCCESS STORIES
AND TESTIMONIALS

Real-Life Experiences of Individuals
Who Have Followed the Pritikin Diet

The Pritikin Diet has garnered numerous success stories from individuals who have embraced its principles and made positive changes to their health and well-being. Here are a few real-life experiences of people who have followed the Pritikin Diet:

1. **John's Weight Loss Journey:** John struggled with obesity and high blood pressure. After adopting the Pritikin Diet, he lost over 50 pounds and saw significant improvements in his blood pressure readings. He attributes his success to the emphasis on whole, unprocessed foods and portion control.

2. **Sara's Cholesterol Reduction:** Sara had high cholesterol levels and a family history of heart disease. Following the Pritikin Diet helped her lower her cholesterol levels and improve her

overall heart health. She found the variety of fruits, vegetables, and whole grains to be satisfying and enjoyable.

3. **Mark's Diabetes Management:** Mark was diagnosed with type 2 diabetes and was determined to manage the condition naturally. By following the Pritikin Diet, he achieved significant weight loss, improved his blood sugar control, and reduced his reliance on diabetes medication. He appreciated the balanced meals and low-glycemic index foods.

Transformation Stories and Health Improvements

The Pritikin Diet has been associated with various health improvements and transformative experiences. Here are some common areas where individuals have witnessed positive changes:

1. **Weight Loss:** Many individuals have successfully lost weight and maintained a healthy weight by following the Pritikin Diet. The focus on whole, nutrient-dense foods and portion control helps create a calorie deficit, leading to sustainable weight loss.

2. **Improved Cardiovascular Health:** The Pritikin Diet's emphasis on low-sodium, low-saturated fat, and cholesterol-lowering foods has resulted in improved cardiovascular health for many individuals. They have seen reductions in blood

pressure, cholesterol levels, and a decreased risk of heart disease.

3. **Better Blood Sugar Control:** People with type 2 diabetes or prediabetes have experienced improved blood sugar control by adopting the Pritikin Diet. The diet's low-glycemic index foods, emphasis on fiber-rich carbohydrates, and portion control contribute to better glucose management.

4. **Increased Energy Levels:** Many individuals have reported increased energy levels and improved overall vitality while following the Pritikin Diet. Nutrient-dense foods and regular physical activity synergistically contribute to enhanced energy and well-being.

5. **Enhanced Mental Well-being:** Some individuals have noticed improvements in their mental health, including reduced stress levels, improved mood, and better cognitive function. The combination of a balanced diet, regular exercise, and healthy lifestyle practices can have a positive impact on mental well-being.

Tips and Advice from Successful Pritikin Diet Followers

Here are some tips and advice from successful individuals who have embraced the Pritikin Diet:

1. **Start Small and Be Consistent:** Begin by making small changes to your diet and lifestyle. Gradually incorporate more whole, unprocessed foods into

your meals and find physical activities you enjoy. Consistency is key to long-term success.

2. **Embrace the Power of Plants:** Focus on increasing your intake of fruits, vegetables, whole grains, legumes, and other plant-based foods. They provide essential nutrients, fiber, and antioxidants that support overall health.

3. **Experiment with Recipes:** Explore new recipes and cooking techniques that incorporate Pritikin Diet principles. It helps keep your meals exciting and diverse, preventing boredom and increasing adherence to the diet.

4. **Stay Hydrated:** Drink plenty of water throughout the day to support optimal hydration. Hydration is important for overall health and can help curb unnecessary food cravings.

5. **Stay Active:** Engage in regular physical activity to complement the Pritikin Diet. Find activities you enjoy, whether it's walking, swimming, cycling, or dancing. Aim for at least 150 minutes of moderate-intensity exercise per week.

6. **Seek Support:** Surround yourself with a supportive network of family, friends, or online communities who are also following the Pritikin Diet. Sharing experiences, recipes, and challenges can provide encouragement and motivation.

7. **Monitor Progress and Celebrate Milestones:** Keep track of your progress by regularly monitoring key health markers such as weight, blood pressure, cholesterol levels, and blood sugar levels. Celebrate milestones and achievements

along the way to stay motivated.

Remember, everyone's journey is unique, and it's essential to listen to your body and make adjustments that work for you. The Pritikin Diet is a long-term commitment to health, and adopting a positive mindset and sustainable habits are crucial for success.

PRITIKIN DIET RECIPES

Hearty Beef and Vegetable Soup

Description: This hearty beef and vegetable soup is a comforting and nutritious meal that will warm you up on a chilly day. Tender chunks of beef are simmered with an array of colourful vegetables, creating a delicious and satisfying broth.

Ingredients:

- 500g beef stew meat, cut into bite-sized pieces
- 2 carrots, peeled and diced
- 2 cclcry stalks, chopped
- 1 onion, finely chopped
- 2 garlic cloves, minced
- 1 can diced tomatoes
- 4 cups beef broth
- 1 bay leaf

- 1 teaspoon dried thyme
- Salt and pepper to taste
- Fresh parsley, chopped (for garnish)

Instructions:

1. In a large pot, heat some olive oil over medium heat. Add the beef and brown it on all sides. Remove the beef from the pot and set it aside.

2. In the same pot, add the carrots, celery, onion, and garlic. Sauté until the vegetables are tender.

3. Return the beef to the pot and add the diced tomatoes, beef broth, bay leaf, dried thyme, salt, and pepper. Stir well.

4. Bring the soup to a boil, then reduce the heat to low and let it simmer for about 1 hour, or until the beef is tender.

5. Remove the bay leaf before serving. Ladle the soup into bowls and garnish with fresh parsley.

Nutritional Information:

- Calories: 250
- Protein: 25g
- Carbohydrates: 20g
- Fat: 8g
- Fiber: 5g

Creamy Chicken and Mushroom Broth

Description: Indulge in the creamy goodness of this

chicken and mushroom broth. This velvety soup combines tender chicken, earthy mushrooms, and a touch of cream for a comforting and satisfying meal.

Ingredients:

- 2 chicken breasts, cooked and shredded
- 200g mushrooms, sliced
- 1 onion, finely chopped
- 2 garlic cloves, minced
- 4 cups chicken broth
- 1 cup heavy cream
- 1 teaspoon dried thyme
- Salt and pepper to taste
- Fresh chives, chopped (for garnish)

Instructions:

1. In a large pot, sauté the mushrooms, onion, and garlic until the mushrooms are golden brown and the onion is translucent.

2. Add the shredded chicken, chicken broth, dried thyme, salt, and pepper to the pot. Stir well.

3. Bring the broth to a boil, then reduce the heat to low and simmer for about 15 minutes to allow the flavors to meld together.

4. Stir in the heavy cream and let the soup simmer for another 5 minutes.

5. Ladle the creamy chicken and mushroom broth

into bowls and garnish with fresh chives.

Nutritional Information:

- Calories: 300
- Protein: 30g
- Carbohydrates: 10g
- Fat: 15g
- Fiber: 2g

Spiced Lentil and Kale Stew

Description: Warm up with a bowl of this spiced lentil and kale stew. Packed with protein-rich lentils, nutrient-dense kale, and aromatic spices, this stew is both comforting and nourishing.

Ingredients:

- 1 cup dried lentils
- 2 tablespoons olive oil
- 1 onion, finely chopped
- 2 carrots, diced
- 2 celery stalks, chopped
- 2 garlic cloves, minced
- 1 teaspoon ground cumin
- 1 teaspoon ground coriander
- 1/2 teaspoon turmeric
- 4 cups vegetable broth

- 2 cups chopped kale
- Salt and pepper to taste
- Fresh cilantro, chopped (for garnish)

Instructions:

1. Rinse the lentils under cold water and set them aside.

2. Heat the olive oil in a large pot over medium heat. Add the onion, carrots, celery, and garlic. Sauté until the vegetables are softened.

3. Stir in the cumin, coriander, and turmeric. Cook for another minute to toast the spices.

4. Add the lentils and vegetable broth to the pot. Bring to a boil, then reduce the heat and simmer for about 20 minutes, or until the lentils are tender.

5. Stir in the chopped kale and cook for an additional 5 minutes until wilted.

6. Season with salt and pepper to taste. Serve the spiced lentil and kale stew in bowls, garnished with fresh cilantro.

Nutritional Information:

- Calories: 220
- Protein: 15g
- Carbohydrates: 35g
- Fat: 5g
- Fiber: 10g

Roasted Turkey Bone Broth

Description: Utilize the full potential of a roasted turkey by making this flavourful bone broth. Simmered with aromatic herbs and vegetables, this broth is a versatile base for many dishes or a soothing, nutritious drink on its own.

Ingredients:

- 1 roasted turkey carcass
- 2 carrots, roughly chopped
- 2 celery stalks, roughly chopped
- 1 onion, quartered
- 4 cloves garlic
- 2 bay leaves
- 1 tablespoon whole peppercorns
- Handful of fresh parsley
- Water (enough to cover the turkey carcass)
- Salt to taste

Instructions:

1. Place the roasted turkey carcass in a large stockpot.
2. Add the carrots, celery, onion, garlic, bay leaves, peppercorns, and parsley to the pot.
3. Pour enough water into the pot to cover the turkey carcass.

4. Bring the mixture to a boil, then reduce the heat to low and simmer for at least 6 hours, or up to 24 hours for a richer flavor.

5. Skim off any foam or impurities that rise to the surface during simmering.

6. After simmering, strain the broth through a fine-mesh sieve into another pot or large bowl.

7. Discard the solids and season the broth with salt to taste.

8. Use the roasted turkey bone broth as a base for soups, stews, or as a comforting drink.

Nutritional Information:

- Calories: 40
- Protein: 5g
- Carbohydrates: 5g
- Fat: 1g
- Fiber: 1g

Ginger and Garlic Infused Fish Soup

Description: Dive into the refreshing flavors of this ginger and garlic infused fish soup. Made with delicate white fish, aromatic spices, and a hint of citrus, this soup is light, fragrant, and perfect for seafood lovers.

Ingredients:

- 500g white fish fillets, cut into bite-sized pieces

- 1 tablespoon olive oil
- 1 onion, finely chopped
- 2 garlic cloves, minced
- 1 tablespoon grated ginger
- 4 cups fish or vegetable broth
- 1 can coconut milk
- Zest and juice of 1 lime
- Fresh cilantro, chopped (for garnish)
- Red chili flakes (optional, for added heat)
- Salt and pepper to taste

Instructions:

1. Heat the olive oil in a large pot over medium heat. Add the onion, garlic, and grated ginger. Sauté until fragrant and the onion is translucent.

2. Add the fish fillets to the pot and cook for a few minutes until they start to turn opaque.

3. Pour in the fish or vegetable broth and bring to a simmer. Let it cook for about 10 minutes.

4. Stir in the coconut milk, lime zest, and lime juice. Season with salt, pepper, and red chili flakes if desired. Simmer for an additional 5 minutes.

5. Ladle the ginger and garlic infused fish soup into bowls and garnish with fresh cilantro.

6. Serve hot and enjoy the delicate flavors.

Nutritional Information:

- Calories: 280

- Protein: 25g
- Carbohydrates: 6g
- Fat: 18g
- Fiber: 1g

Nourishing Vegetable and Quinoa Broth

Description: This nourishing vegetable and quinoa broth is a wholesome and satisfying meal in a bowl. Packed with colourful vegetables, protein-rich quinoa, and aromatic herbs, it provides a boost of nutrients to keep you energized.

Ingredients:

- 1 tablespoon olive oil
- 1 onion, finely chopped
- 2 carrots, diced
- 2 celery stalks, chopped
- 1 bell pepper, diced
- 2 garlic cloves, minced
- 1 teaspoon dried thyme
- 1 teaspoon dried oregano
- 1/2 cup quinoa
- 4 cups vegetable broth
- Salt and pepper to taste
- Fresh parsley, chopped (for garnish)

Instructions:

1. Heat the olive oil in a large pot over medium heat. Add the onion, carrots, celery, bell pepper, and garlic. Sauté until the vegetables are tender.

2. Stir in the dried thyme, dried oregano, and quinoa. Cook for a minute to toast the quinoa and release the flavors.

3. Pour in the vegetable broth and bring the mixture to a boil. Reduce the heat and let it simmer for about 15-20 minutes, or until the quinoa is cooked and the vegetables are soft.

4. Season with salt and pepper to taste.

5. Ladle the nourishing vegetable and quinoa broth into bowls and garnish with fresh parsley.

6. Serve hot and enjoy the wholesome goodness.

Nutritional Information:

- Calories: 220
- Protein: 7g
- Carbohydrates: 40g
- Fat: 5g
- Fiber: 8g

Fragrant Thai Coconut Chicken Soup

Description: Immerse yourself in the aromatic and exotic flavors of this fragrant Thai coconut chicken soup. With tender chicken, vibrant vegetables, and a blend of Thai spices, this soup is a delightful balance of sweet, spicy, and tangy notes.

Ingredients:

- 2 chicken breasts, thinly sliced
- 1 tablespoon vegetable oil
- 1 onion, finely chopped
- 2 garlic cloves, minced
- 1 red bell pepper, sliced
- 1 zucchini, sliced
- 1 can coconut milk
- 4 cups chicken broth
- 2 tablespoons Thai red curry paste
- 1 tablespoon fish sauce
- 1 tablespoon brown sugar
- Juice of 1 lime
- Fresh cilantro, chopped (for garnish)
- Red chili flakes (optional, for added heat)
- Salt and pepper to taste

Instructions:

1. Heat the vegetable oil in a large pot over medium heat. Add the onion, garlic, and red bell pepper. Sauté until the vegetables are softened.
2. Add the chicken slices to the pot and cook until they are no longer pink.

3. Stir in the Thai red curry paste and cook for a minute to release its flavors.

4. Pour in the coconut milk and chicken broth. Bring the mixture to a simmer.

5. Add the zucchini slices, fish sauce, brown sugar, lime juice, salt, and pepper. Simmer for about 10 minutes, or until the vegetables are tender.

6. Adjust the seasoning according to your taste preferences. If desired, add red chili flakes for additional heat.

7. Ladle the fragrant Thai coconut chicken soup into bowls and garnish with fresh cilantro.

8. Serve hot and enjoy the exotic Thai flavors.

Nutritional Information:

- Calories: 320
- Protein: 25g
- Carbohydrates: 15g
- Fat: 20g
- Fiber: 3g

Savory Lamb and Barley Stew

Description: Experience the rich and hearty flavors of this savory lamb and barley stew. Slow-cooked to perfection, this stew features tender lamb, wholesome barley, and a medley of vegetables, creating a satisfying and comforting meal.

Ingredients:

- 500g lamb stew meat, cut into chunks
- 2 tablespoons olive oil
- 1 onion, finely chopped
- 2 carrots, diced
- 2 celery stalks, chopped
- 2 garlic cloves, minced
- 1 can diced tomatoes
- 4 cups beef or vegetable broth
- 1/2 cup pearl barley
- 1 teaspoon dried rosemary
- 1 teaspoon dried thyme
- Salt and pepper to taste
- Fresh parsley, chopped (for garnish)

Instructions:

1. Heat the olive oil in a large pot over medium heat. Add the lamb chunks and cook until browned on all sides. Remove the lamb from the pot and set it aside.

2. In the same pot, add the onion, carrots, celery, and garlic. Sauté until the vegetables are softened.

3. Return the lamb to the pot and add the diced tomatoes, broth, pearl barley, dried rosemary, dried thyme, salt, and pepper. Stir well.

4. Bring the stew to a boil, then reduce the heat to low and let it simmer for about 1.5 to 2 hours, or

until the lamb is tender and the barley is cooked.

5. Adjust the seasoning if needed.

6. Ladle the savory lamb and barley stew into bowls and garnish with fresh parsley.

7. Serve hot and enjoy the comforting flavors.

Nutritional Information:

- Calories: 380
- Protein: 30g
- Carbohydrates: 20g
- Fat: 18g
- Fiber: 4g

Roasted Cauliflower and Turmeric Broth

Description: Indulge in the comforting and vibrant flavors of this roasted cauliflower and turmeric broth. Roasted cauliflower adds depth and nuttiness to this broth, while the warm and earthy notes of turmeric create a soothing and aromatic experience.

Ingredients:

- 1 medium cauliflower, cut into florets
- 2 tablespoons olive oil
- 1 onion, finely chopped
- 2 cloves garlic, minced
- 1 teaspoon ground turmeric

- 4 cups vegetable broth
- 1 can coconut milk
- Juice of 1 lemon
- Salt and pepper to taste
- Fresh coriander, chopped (for garnish)

Instructions:

1. Preheat the oven to 200°C (400°F). Place the cauliflower florets on a baking sheet and drizzle with olive oil. Season with salt and pepper. Roast in the oven for about 20 minutes, or until the cauliflower is tender and golden brown.

2. In a large pot, heat olive oil over medium heat. Add the chopped onion and minced garlic. Sauté until the onion becomes translucent and fragrant.

3. Stir in the ground turmeric and cook for a minute to release its flavors.

4. Add the roasted cauliflower florets to the pot, followed by the vegetable broth and coconut milk. Bring the mixture to a simmer and let it cook for about 10 minutes.

5. Using an immersion blender or a regular blender, blend the soup until smooth and creamy.

6. Stir in the lemon juice and season with salt and pepper according to your taste.

7. Ladle the roasted cauliflower and turmeric broth into bowls and garnish with fresh coriander.

8. Serve hot and enjoy the comforting and nourishing flavors.

Nutritional Information:

- Calories: 220
- Protein: 6g
- Carbohydrates: 14g
- Fat: 18g
- Fiber: 4g

Smoky Tomato and White Bean Soup

Description: Delight in the smoky and comforting flavors of this tomato and white bean soup. With the combination of sweet tomatoes, creamy white beans, and a touch of smokiness, this soup is a satisfying and hearty option for any occasion.

Ingredients:

- 2 tablespoons olive oil
- 1 onion, finely chopped
- 2 cloves garlic, minced
- 1 teaspoon smoked paprika
- 1/2 teaspoon cumin
- 1 can diced tomatoes
- 4 cups vegetable broth
- 1 can white beans, drained and rinsed
- 1 bay leaf

- Salt and pepper to taste
- Fresh parsley, chopped (for garnish)

Instructions:

1. Heat olive oil in a large pot over medium heat. Add the chopped onion and minced garlic. Sauté until the onion becomes translucent and fragrant.

2. Stir in the smoked paprika and cumin, and cook for a minute to toast the spices.

3. Add the diced tomatoes, vegetable broth, white beans, and bay leaf to the pot. Stir well to combine.

4. Bring the mixture to a boil, then reduce the heat and let it simmer for about 15-20 minutes, allowing the flavors to meld together.

5. Remove the bay leaf from the soup and discard.

6. Using an immersion blender or a regular blender, blend a portion of the soup to achieve a partially smooth texture while leaving some chunks for added texture.

7. Season with salt and pepper to taste.

8. Ladle the smoky tomato and white bean soup into bowls and garnish with fresh parsley.

9. Serve hot and savour the delicious and comforting flavours.

Nutritional Information:

- Calories: 210
- Protein: 8g

- Carbohydrates: 30g
- Fat: 6g
- Fiber: 8g

Tangy Shrimp and Lime Broth

Description: Immerse your taste buds in the zesty and tangy flavours of this shrimp and lime broth. Succulent shrimp, fresh vegetables, and a burst of lime juice create a light and refreshing soup that is perfect for a light meal or starter.

Ingredients:

- 500g shrimp, peeled and deveined
- 1 tablespoon vegetable oil
- 1 onion, finely chopped
- 2 cloves garlic, minced
- 1 red bell pepper, thinly sliced
- 1 carrot, julienned
- 4 cups fish or vegetable broth
- Juice of 2 limes
- 1 tablespoon soy sauce
- 1 tablespoon fish sauce
- Fresh coriander, chopped (for garnish)
- Red chili flakes (optional, for added heat)
- Salt and pepper to taste

Instructions:

1. Heat the vegetable oil in a large pot over medium heat. Add the chopped onion and minced garlic. Sauté until the onion becomes translucent and fragrant.

2. Add the shrimp to the pot and cook until they turn pink and opaque. Remove the shrimp from the pot and set aside.

3. In the same pot, add the red bell pepper and carrot. Sauté for a few minutes until slightly tender.

4. Pour in the fish or vegetable broth, lime juice, soy sauce, and fish sauce. Bring the broth to a simmer.

5. Season with salt, pepper, and red chili flakes if desired. Simmer for about 10 minutes to allow the flavours to meld together.

6. Return the cooked shrimp to the pot and cook for an additional 2-3 minutes to heat through.

7. Ladle the tangy shrimp and lime broth into bowls and garnish with fresh coriander.

8. Serve hot and savour the zesty and tangy flavours.

Nutritional Information:

- Calories: 220
- Protein: 25g
- Carbohydrates: 9g
- Fat: 8g
- Fiber: 2g

Herbed Chicken and Sweet Potato Stew

Description: Warm your soul with the comforting and aromatic flavours of this herbed chicken and sweet potato stew. Tender chicken, hearty sweet potatoes, and a blend of fragrant herbs create a hearty and satisfying meal that will leave you feeling nourished.

Ingredients:

- 500g chicken thighs, boneless and skinless, cut into chunks
- 2 tablespoons olive oil
- 1 onion, finely chopped
- 2 cloves garlic, minced
- 2 carrots, diced
- 2 sweet potatoes, peeled and diced
- 4 cups chicken broth
- 1 teaspoon dried thyme
- 1 teaspoon dried rosemary
- 1 bay leaf
- Salt and pepper to taste
- Fresh parsley, chopped (for garnish)

Instructions:

1. Heat the olive oil in a large pot over medium heat. Add the chopped onion and minced garlic. Sauté

until the onion becomes translucent and fragrant.

2. Add the chicken chunks to the pot and cook until they are browned on all sides.

3. Stir in the diced carrots, sweet potatoes, chicken broth, dried thyme, dried rosemary, bay leaf, salt, and pepper. Bring the stew to a boil.

4. Reduce the heat to low, cover the pot, and let the stew simmer for about 30-40 minutes, or until the chicken is cooked through and the sweet potatoes are tender.

5. Remove the bay leaf from the stew and discard.

6. Adjust the seasoning if needed.

7. Ladle the herbed chicken and sweet potato stew into bowls and garnish with fresh parsley.

8. Serve hot and enjoy the comforting and nourishing flavours.

Nutritional Information:

- Calories: 320
- Protein: 25g
- Carbohydrates: 25g
- Fat: 12g
- Fiber: 4g

Tomato Basil Bisque with Bone Broth

Description: Indulge in the creamy and rich flavours of this tomato basil bisque with bone broth. Velvety smooth and packed with the essence of ripe tomatoes and aromatic basil, this soup is a comforting and satisfying treat for your taste buds.

Ingredients:

- 2 tablespoons butter
- 1 onion, finely chopped
- 2 cloves garlic, minced
- 2 cans diced tomatoes
- 4 cups bone broth
- 1/2 cup heavy cream
- Handful of fresh basil leaves, chopped
- Salt and pepper to taste
- Grated Parmesan cheese (for garnish)

Instructions:

1. In a large pot, melt the butter over medium heat. Add the chopped onion and minced garlic. Sauté until the onion becomes translucent and fragrant.
2. Add the diced tomatoes (with their juice) to the pot. Stir well to combine.
3. Pour in the bone broth and bring the mixture to a simmer. Let it cook for about 15-20 minutes to allow the flavours to meld together.
4. Using an immersion blender or a regular blender, blend the soup until smooth and creamy.
5. Return the blended soup to the pot and stir in the heavy cream and chopped basil leaves. Season

with salt and pepper according to your taste.

6. Heat the soup over low heat for an additional 5 minutes to warm it through.

7. Ladle the tomato basil bisque into bowls and garnish with grated Parmesan cheese.

8. Serve hot and savour the creamy and comforting flavours.

Nutritional Information:

- Calories: 230

- Protein: 10g

- Carbohydrates: 15g

- Fat: 15g

- Fiber: 4g

Vegetarian Chickpea and Spinach Soup

Description: Delight in the hearty and nutritious flavours of this vegetarian chickpea and spinach soup. Packed with protein-rich chickpeas, vibrant spinach, and a blend of aromatic spices, this soup is a satisfying and wholesome choice for vegetarians and vegans.

Ingredients:

- 2 tablespoons olive oil

- 1 onion, finely chopped

- 2 cloves garlic, minced

- 1 carrot, diced
- 2 celery stalks, chopped
- 1 can chickpeas, drained and rinsed
- 4 cups vegetable broth
- 2 cups fresh spinach leaves
- 1 teaspoon ground cumin
- 1/2 teaspoon ground coriander
- 1/2 teaspoon paprika
- Salt and pepper to taste
- Fresh parsley, chopped (for garnish)

Instructions:

1. Heat the olive oil in a large pot over medium heat. Add the chopped onion and minced garlic. Sauté until the onion becomes translucent and fragrant.

2. Add the diced carrot, chopped celery, and drained chickpeas to the pot. Stir well to combine.

3. Pour in the vegetable broth and bring the mixture to a boil. Reduce the heat and let it simmer for about 15-20 minutes, or until the vegetables are tender.

4. Add the fresh spinach leaves to the pot and stir until wilted.

5. Stir in the ground cumin, ground coriander, paprika, salt, and pepper. Simmer for an additional 5 minutes to allow the flavours to meld together.

6. Adjust the seasoning if needed.

7. Ladle the vegetarian chickpea and spinach soup into bowls and garnish with fresh parsley.

8. Serve hot and enjoy the hearty and nutritious flavours.

Nutritional Information:

- Calories: 210

- Protein: 9g

- Carbohydrates: 30g

- Fat: 7g

- Fiber: 8g

Mexican-inspired Beef and Black Bean Broth

Description: Embark on a culinary journey with the vibrant and flavourful Mexican-inspired beef and black bean broth. Tender beef, hearty black beans, and a medley of aromatic spices create a savoury and satisfying soup that will transport you to the streets of Mexico.

Ingredients:

- 500g beef stew meat, cubed

- 2 tablespoons olive oil

- 1 onion, finely chopped

- 2 cloves garlic, minced

- 1 red bell pepper, diced

- 1 can black beans, drained and rinsed

- 4 cups beef broth
- 1 teaspoon ground cumin
- 1/2 teaspoon chili powder
- 1/2 teaspoon paprika
- Juice of 1 lime
- Salt and pepper to taste
- Fresh coriander, chopped (for garnish)
- Avocado slices (for garnish)
- Tortilla chips (for serving)

Instructions:

1. Heat the olive oil in a large pot over medium heat. Add the cubed beef stew meat and cook until browned on all sides. Remove the beef from the pot and set aside.

2. In the same pot, add the chopped onion, minced garlic, and diced red bell pepper. Sauté until the onion becomes translucent and fragrant.

3. Return the cooked beef to the pot and add the black beans, beef broth, ground cumin, chili powder, and paprika. Stir well to combine.

4. Bring the broth to a boil, then reduce the heat and let it simmer for about 1 to 1.5 hours, or until the beef is tender.

5. Stir in the lime juice and season with salt and pepper according to your taste.

6. Ladle the Mexican-inspired beef and black bean broth into bowls.

7. Garnish with fresh coriander and avocado slices.

8. Serve hot with tortilla chips for a crunchy texture.

Nutritional Information:

- Calories: 320
- Protein: 26g
- Carbohydrates: 18g
- Fat: 16g
- Fiber: 6g

CONCLUSION

Recap of Key Points Discussed

Throughout the Ebook

Throughout this ebook, we have explored various aspects of the Pritikin Diet and its potential impact on health and well-being. Here's a recap of the key points discussed:

1. The Pritikin Diet is a whole-food, plant-based eating plan that emphasizes low-sodium, low-saturated fat, and cholesterol-lowering foods.

2. The diet is based on the principles of consuming nutrient-dense foods, focusing on whole grains, fruits, vegetables, lean proteins, and healthy fats.

3. The Pritikin Diet is rooted in scientific research and has been associated with numerous health benefits, including weight loss, improved cardiovascular health, better blood sugar control, increased energy levels, and enhanced mental well-being.

4. Key components of the diet include high-fiber foods, whole grains, lean proteins, and healthy fats.

5. Portion control is essential to maintain a healthy caloric intake and achieve weight management

goals.

6. The diet encourages incorporating a wide variety of fruits and vegetables into daily meals.

7. Sample meal plans for breakfast, lunch, and dinner, as well as snack ideas, were provided to give readers practical guidance.

8. Strategies for dining out, travelling, and meal prepping while on the Pritikin Diet were discussed to help readers navigate real-life situations.

9. The Pritikin Diet supports weight loss through its focus on whole, nutrient-dense foods and portion control.

10. Strategies for portion control and mindful eating were outlined to help readers develop healthy eating habits.

11. Regular physical activity is recommended to complement the Pritikin Diet for optimal health benefits.

12. Monitoring progress, setting realistic goals, and seeking professional guidance were emphasized to track and maintain success.

13. Strategies for overcoming cravings, managing hunger, and dealing with social situations while following the Pritikin Diet were provided.

14. The importance of adjusting the diet for specific health conditions and considering nutrient deficiencies and supplementation was discussed.

15. Stress management, the importance of sleep, and strategies for long-term adherence to the Pritikin

Diet were explored.

Encouragement and Motivation to Try the Pritikin Diet

If you're considering trying the Pritikin Diet, it's important to remember that making positive changes to your eating habits and lifestyle is a journey. The Pritikin Diet offers a scientifically backed approach to improving your health and well-being. By embracing its principles and incorporating them into your daily life, you have the potential to experience numerous benefits, including weight loss, improved cardiovascular health, better blood sugar control, increased energy levels, and enhanced mental well-being.

It's important to approach the diet with an open mind and a willingness to make sustainable changes. Start by gradually incorporating more whole, unprocessed foods into your meals and finding physical activities that you enjoy. Seek support from friends, family, or online communities who are also following the Pritikin Diet to share experiences and gain motivation. Remember that every step you take towards a healthier lifestyle is a step in the right direction.

Final Thoughts on the Potential Impact of the Pritikin Diet on Health and Well-being

The Pritikin Diet offers a holistic approach to improving health and well-being through its emphasis on whole, nutrient-dense foods and lifestyle modifications. By adopting this eating plan, individuals have the opportunity to achieve weight loss, improve cardiovascular health, manage blood sugar levels, increase energy, and enhance mental well-being.

The diet's focus on high-fiber foods, whole grains, lean proteins, and healthy fats provides essential nutrients while reducing the intake of sodium, saturated fat, and cholesterol. These dietary modifications, coupled with portion control and regular physical activity, can have a profound impact on overall health and quality of life.

While the Pritikin Diet may require adjustments and initial commitment, the potential benefits make it worth considering for those seeking to improve their health and make sustainable lifestyle changes. By adopting this approach to eating and incorporating the principles into your daily life, you can take charge of your well-being and enjoy the positive effects it may bring.

Remember, consult with a healthcare professional before making any significant dietary changes, especially if you have underlying health conditions or are on medication. They can provide personalised guidance and support based on your individual needs and help you navigate the journey towards improved health and well-being.